Before and After
Radical
Prostate
Surgery

Information and Resource Guide

Virginia Vandall-Walker RN PhD
with Katherine Moore RN PhD and Diane Pyne RN MHS

AU PRESS

© 2008 Virginia Vandall-Walker, Katherine Moore, Diane Pyne

Published by **AU Press,**
Athabasca University
1200, 10011 - 109 Street
Edmonton, AB T5J 3S8

Library and Archives Canada Cataloguing in Publication

Vandall-Walker, Virginia, 1950–
Before and after radical prostate surgery: information and
resource guide / Virginia Vandall-Walker, Katherine Moore,
Diane Pyne.

Issued also in electronic format.
ISBN 978-1-897425-17-6

1. Prostate–Cancer–Surgery–Popular works.
2. Patient education.
I. Moore, Katherine N. (Katherine Nancy), 1946–
II. Pyne, Diane, 1956–
III. Title.

RD587.V35 2008   616.99'463   C2008-905567-5

Printed and bound in Canada by AGMV Marquis

Cover and book design by Alex Chan/Studio Reface
Illustrations by Dwight Allott

You can order additional copies of this guide online at
www.ubcpress

TABLE OF CONTENTS

INTRODUCTION

Prostate cancer affects one in eight Canadian men, primarily between the ages of 50 and 79. In Canada, over 22,000 new cases are diagnosed every year. Of these men, approximately 20% will undergo prostate surgery. *Before and After Radical Prostate Surgery* provides concise information and management tips that will be useful for men (and their partners) in the hospital and at home, as well as information about new surgical options for prostate cancer that are available in some Canadian centres. This guide is useful as well for those who are still in the process of decision-making about their treatment choices.

The key sources of information for the authors of this guide were men who have undergone radical prostate surgery and some of their partners, as well as health professionals working with men undergoing prostate surgery. The participants in our study related the difficulties and challenges they experienced before making the decision to undergo a radical prostatectomy (RP) as their treatment choice.

Individuals who shared their prostate surgery experiences with us described the importance of support, both individually and where applicable, as a couple, from family, friends, health professionals and their local Prostate Support Group. Men also spoke of the need to be as healthy and fit as possible before going into surgery. Additionally, men and their partners discussed the value of talking openly with each other and with health professionals about the emotional aspects of dealing with the diagnosis of cancer, exploring treatment options, and the surgical and recovery experience. Counseling was found to be very beneficial by those who experienced it.

Because the majority of the men in our study had partners who also chose to participate, we were able to include this important perspective. While not everyone considering or undergoing RP surgery will have a partner or spouse, many men will have a friend or relative sharing the journey, who will also find the information in this guide applicable.

It must be noted that radical prostate surgery is a very individual experience, not least because hospital and surgical procedures vary across the country. Your hospital and your urologist will provide you with the specific information you need. While we urge readers of this guide to seek all available resources to meet their information needs, we suggest that you discuss the information you find with a health professional involved in your care to confirm that it is credible and up-to-date.

We trust that you will find our efforts to be beneficial for you, your partner, and your family.

Virginia Katherine Diane

ACKNOWLEDGEMENTS

This book would not have been possible without the dedication and drive of the men and their partners, urology nurses, and urologists, who volunteered their time to this project. AU Press would like to acknowledge this commitment and sincerely thank these individuals for their determination to bring this important project to fruition.

The authors would particularly like to thank:

Athabasca University's Academic Research Fund
Edmonton Prostate Cancer Support Group
Dr. Eric Estey
Dr. Michael Hobart

This book is endorsed by:

Canadian Prostate Cancer Network/Réseau Canadien du
 cancer de la prostate
The Canadian Continence Foundation
Canadian Urological Association
Urology Nurses of Canada.

BEFORE SURGERY, AT HOME

Who is a Candidate for Radical Prostate Surgery?

Men who have prostate cancer are candidates for radical prostate surgery when the tumour is localized in the prostate gland and the cancer has not spread beyond the prostate gland.

What is a Radical Retropubic Prostatectomy?

The prostate gland is one of the organs that secrete a fluid that mixes with sperm to make semen. This gland lies deep in the pelvis behind the pubic bone and surrounds the urethra, which is the tube that carries urine from the bladder to the penis.

A radical retropubic prostatectomy is surgery to remove the prostate gland, the seminal vesicles (that produce fluid for semen), and the part of the urethra that passes through the prostate. In some cases, lymph nodes in the area surrounding the prostate gland may also be removed, as well as one or both of the nerve bundles adjoining the prostate gland. The decision on how extensive the surgery should be, which depends on the individual situation, is determined during surgery. The relevant parts of the body are identified in the diagram below.

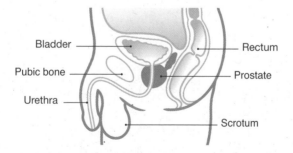

The Types of Procedures Used

There are a number of ways to remove the prostate gland. Some procedures you may have heard about are no longer performed. It is important to discuss and understand the procedure that your urologist will be using for your own surgery. This guide focuses on three procedures for performing a radical retropubic prostatectomy, which is the complete removal of the prostate gland through an incision or incisions made in the abdomen to access the gland lying behind the pubic bone.

1. The "open procedure"

The traditional surgery for prostate cancer is known as the "open procedure." A catheter is inserted into the bladder through the urethra to help stabilize the urethra during the procedure. The surgeon then opens an incision 8 to 10 centimetres long in the patient's abdomen from the belly-button to the pubic bone through which the prostate gland and a small part of the urethra are then removed. Other adjacent organs may also be removed. The cut end of the urethra is then sewn to the neck of the bladder. Drains are placed around the surgical site and then the incision is closed (see Fig. 1).

2. The laparoscopic procedure

The term "laparoscopy" refers to a surgical technique in which a lighted viewing instrument with a camera (laparoscope) is inserted into the lower belly through a port placed into a small incision made below the navel. The laparoscope is a long, thin, flexible tube used to guide the operation. Carbon dioxide (CO_2) put into the abdomen through a special needle helps to separate the organs inside the abdominal cavity from the abdominal wall, making it easier for the surgeon to see and remove the prostate gland. This gas is removed at the end of the procedure. The surgeon then uses four other incision sites, usually no longer than 5 millimetres, for the introduction of instruments to cut and remove the prostate gland. This procedure is frequently referred to as the "lap procedure" (see Fig. 2).

3. The robotic laparoscopic procedure

The third procedure used for radical retropubic prostatectomy is referred to as the "robotic lap." The operation uses the same techniques and incision sites as described for a "lap"; however, the surgeon performs the technique by controlling a robot, called the "Da Vinci Robot." Both the robot and the procedure are frequently referred to by the term "robo" (see Fig. 2).

Research has demonstrated that all three of these procedures are equally effective for removing the prostate gland and surrounding tissues, and for cancer control. Potential side effects, such as incontinence and impotence, are the same for all three procedures. It is important to discuss and understand the method that your urologist will use for your surgery. No matter which procedure is chosen, a radical retropubic prostatectomy may take from 2 to 4 hours to perform using a general anaesthetic to put you to sleep. The side effects of the surgery will vary in severity and duration.

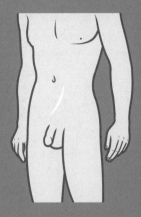

Fig. 1 "Open" Prostatectomy Incision

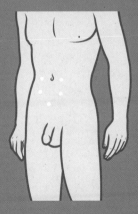

Fig. 2 Laparoscopic and "robo"
Prostatectomy Incisions

Feelings Men and their Partners May Have Before Surgery

A diagnosis of prostate cancer is a shock. We want to reassure you that some of these feelings and mood swings are to be expected.

We encourage you to share your feelings and concerns with your partner and family. They may very well have the same feelings but were afraid to discuss them because they didn't want to worry you. On the other hand, well-meaning family members and friends might try to convince you that you should have a different therapy, or none at all. Listen, but make it clear that the decision is yours to make.

Different people can provide you with different levels and types of support. Be sure to discuss your feelings with your urologist, urology nurse, or your family physician. Your local Prostate Cancer Support Group can offer information and an opportunity to talk to men and their partners who have been through prostate surgery and other treatments. Many men reported finding counseling very helpful. Most cancer hospitals have psychologists who are available to you and your family. As well, the Canadian Prostate Cancer Network (CPCN) has up-to-date information on support groups and therapists near you. Call 1-866-810-2726 or visit the website at *www.cpcn.org*.

- **Disbelief** *This can't be!*

- **Anger (sometimes targeted at a partner)** *Why me? How could this happen?*

- **Betrayal** *My body has let me down.*

- **Fear of the cancer** *Will it spread? How long do I have to live?*

- **Fear of surgery** *What will they find when they open me up? Will I wake up? Will I regain a sex life?*

- **Loss of control** *My "living" is out of my control!*

- **Uncertainty, confusion** *Have I made the correct treatment decision? Should I choose a different one?*

- **Frustration** *Waiting even one day for surgery is too long!*
  (In most cases, waiting will not affect the outcome of surgery. Talk to your surgeon about this.)

- **Mood swings** *Is this normal? I can't help it!*

What Can You Do While Waiting?

1. Gather Information

- Talk to your urologist. Ask questions. A list of possible questions that you or your partner might have is given on page 16.

- Read! Your local cancer facility will have a library you can access. This guide includes a list of recommended reading on the topic.

- Search the Internet. Some recommended Canadian websites are listed at the end of this guide. (Be aware that some websites are simply advertisements for one therapy or another.)

- Talk about what you have read with your partner, family, urologist, and other members of your health care team.

- Talk to men who have had prostate surgery.

- Attend a Prostate Cancer Support Group meeting in your area. (Family members or close friends are welcome.)

2. Adopt a Healthy Diet and Lifestyle

- Make extra efforts to eat a healthy diet.

- Lose excess weight to help improve your overall health.

- If you smoke, quit.

- Exercise to help with relaxation, weight loss, and tension relief, and to influence positive outcomes after surgery. If you do not now exercise regularly, discuss an exercise program with your family physician or nurse, and then carry it out.

○ Relieve stress by doing things that help you to relax, such as listening to music, having a massage, meditating, or finding opportunities for laughter.

3. Take a Break

○ Take a break from your routine, if you can, such as a vacation.

○ Check with your urologist about your plans to ensure you don't miss appointments.

4. Collect a Few Items for the Recovery Period

Men who have undergone prostate surgery suggest that the following items are useful to have for after your surgery.

○ Loose fitting trousers or sweat pants for comfort over your abdomen

○ A comfortable chair (e.g., a recliner)

○ A soft pillow to make sitting on any chair more comfortable

○ Men's incontinence pads (After surgery, most men have some loss of bladder control.)

○ A few protective pads for the bed, chair, and seat of the car. (Not all men need these.)

○ Look in the Yellow Pages under "Health Care Supplies." At the store, ask for samples so you can choose the product that is best for you. There are many styles of pads good for different amounts of urine loss.

○ See the Canadian Continence Foundation's resource guide at *http://www.canadiancontinence.ca*

5. Practice Pelvic Floor Exercises (see next page)

- Following surgery, you may have trouble controlling your urine.

- The layers of pelvic muscles are like a hammock that helps support your bladder and bowel to prevent leakage of urine and stool. Exercising these muscles may help with urine control after surgery.

- It is best to start practicing these exercises before your surgery.

Pelvic Floor Muscle Exercises

You may do the exercises sitting, standing, or lying down.

Imagine you are trying to stop yourself from passing gas by squeezing the muscle around your anus. You should feel the anus muscle move while the buttocks, thighs, and stomach stay relaxed (without moving).

If you are doing the exercise correctly, you should be able to feel, and if you look, to see, the base of your penis twitch and contract inwards.

⇨ *SQUEEZE firmly for 5 to 10 seconds.*
⇨ *RELAX for 10 to 20 seconds.*
⇨ *REPEAT the contractions 12 to 20 times.*
⇨ *Do the exercises 3 times a day.*

The exercises are easy. If you find it difficult to isolate find the right muscles, a physiotherapist or nurse who specializes in these exercises can explain how to do them correctly. Ask your health professional for information about who provides this service in your area. The nearest Prostate Cancer Support Group may have audiovisual materials in various formats to help you learn how to do these exercises.

Suggested Questions for You and Your Partner to Ask Your Urologist

Remember, it is your body. You want to be as informed as you can be.

- ❑ What is my PSA? What does this mean?
- ❑ What is my Gleason Score? What does this mean?
- ❑ What is my "risk stratification"? What does this mean?
- ❑ What is the approximate weight of my prostate gland in ounces? What does this mean?
- ❑ Where is the tumor located in my prostate gland? What does this mean?
- ❑ Should I donate my own blood before surgery?
- ❑ What type of prostate surgery do you usually perform?
- ❑ How often do you do this surgery?
- ❑ How many hours will I be at the Pre-Admission Clinic?
- ❑ How long will I be in hospital after the surgery?
- ❑ What can I expect about bladder control after surgery?
- ❑ How does the surgery affect erections and sexual activity?
- ❑ Can you tell me more about the nerve sparing procedure?
- ❑ Could you direct me to resources and professionals I can speak to for more information about the procedure?

You or your partner may have other questions.

- ☐ _____
- ☐ _____
- ☐ _____
- ☐ _____
- ☐ _____
- ☐ _____
- ☐ _____
- ☐ _____
- ☐ _____
- ☐ _____
- ☐ _____
- ☐ _____
- ☐ _____
- ☐ _____
- ☐ _____
- ☐ _____
- ☐ _____
- ☐ _____

BEFORE SURGERY, IN HOSPITAL

The Pre-Admission Clinic

Before surgery, personnel from the hospital where you will be having your surgery will call to schedule a time to attend the Pre-Admission Clinic. The timing of the information session before the actual date of your surgery can vary greatly. Prepare for the clinic by reading and talking to health professionals beforehand, as the Pre-Admission Clinic is a very busy time.

We recommend that you bring a family member or friend with you. He or she can help you to remember all the information the clinic staff will provide. At the clinic, you will be told about your specific surgery. Physicians (anaesthetists, residents) and nurses will also ask you for certain information about your health. If you have diabetes, your family physician or urologist may have to change your treatment before your surgery. For example, if you take insulin, you may need to see a diabetic specialist before your surgery.

As any medication can influence what tests you may require, the nurses and physicians will need to know all of the medications you take. For example, ASA (aspirin) and other blood thinners may need to be stopped a week before surgery.

Please make a list of the following information and take it with you to the Pre-Admission Clinic.

❏ Cigarettes (packs per day)

_____

❏ Alcohol (drinks per day)

_____

❏ Herbal medicines (name, dosage)

_____

❏ Non-prescription medications (name, dosage)

_____

❏ Prescription medicines (name, dosage)

_____

_____

THE SURGERY

What You Can Expect

Your Prostatectomy

Your urologist will have explained the specific procedure being performed and what is involved.

When do I go to the hospital for surgery?

The hospital or your urologist's office will let you know what time you should arrive at the hospital.

What "surgical prep" will I have to do?

You will be given specific written instructions about anything you need to do beforehand to prepare for surgery. Most men are asked to use an enema or to take a laxative at home. Some surgeons want you to shower with a special soap before surgery. Some have specific instructions about removing hair on the surgical site.

Anaesthetic

You will be given a sedative before going to the operating room (OR) to relax you. In the OR a general anaesthetic will be administered to put you to sleep for 2 to 4 hours.

Catheter

A catheter is a tube that drains urine from the bladder into a collection bag. It is inserted into the bladder during surgery since your urethra will need to be cut and sutured to the bladder. The catheter is left in place to help drain urine while your urethra is healing (see page 40).

Intravenous (IV)

An IV will be started in the OR, if not before. You will still have the IV when you return to the nursing unit.

AFTER SURGERY, IN HOSPITAL

When Surgery is Over, Then What?

You will wake up in the Post Anaesthetic Care Unit (PACU). You will stay in this unit for 1 to 2 hours. Because of the anaesthetic, you may not remember much about this time. No visitors will be allowed in to see you. Your partner can ask the nurses on your nursing unit about your progress.

Once you are awake, you will go back to a nursing unit. You will feel sleepy and perhaps confused as a result of the anaesthetic, and from the medication given to relieve pain. Nurses will check on your condition frequently. Your friends and relatives may comment that you look pale after the surgery, but your normal colour will return when you start to move around.

You can expect the following:

Oxygen

Oxygen is a standard therapy for a short period after surgery. It is given using either a mask or through small tubes placed in your nose.

Intravenous

You will have an intravenous (IV) line to provide fluid until you are able to drink and eat well. Your medications may also be given through the IV line. IVs should not cause discomfort, so if your IV is painful or very uncomfortable, let your nurse know.

Pain and Discomfort

It is common to have pain and discomfort after surgery. The amount of pain (both incision and gas) and discomfort (catheter and sore throat) will be different from person to person. DO NOT UNDERESTIMATE YOUR PAIN OR DISCOMFORT. Tell your nurse how you feel. She or he will probably assess your pain on a scale of 1 to 10 (with 10 being the worst pain you have ever felt) and will give you medication to control the pain and discomfort.

With good pain control, you will:
- Get well faster.
- Be able to take deep breaths, walk around, and recover strength.
- Avoid problems such as pneumonia and blood clots.

Sore Throat

The tubes used to help you breathe during the operation may cause a sore throat. Your mouth will be dry because you have not had anything to drink for hours. Mouth swabs can help.

Gas Pains

Abdominal gas is very painful. Warm blankets, lying on your left side (if possible), and walking may help to relieve abdominal gas pains. To help prevent gas, don't suck on ice chips. Eat and drink small amounts at a time.

Your Incision(s)

You may have a small drain, perhaps two, in your abdomen to drain fluid. The drain, called a Jackson Pratt, is held in place with stitches, which are usually removed (painlessly) by the time you ready to go home.

If you had an open procedure, you will have one incision in your lower abdomen. Your incision may cause you pain. Holding a pillow over your incision can help to lessen the pain when you move, sneeze, laugh, or cry. Staples may have been used to close the incision. If they are removed in the hospital, the nurse will place steri-strips (small adhesive tapes) over the incision.

If you had a laparoscopic procedure or robotic laparoscopic procedure, you will have four or five small incisions in your abdomen. These small incisions will cause minimal discomfort. Each one will be covered with a Band-Aid or steri-strip.

Catheter Discomfort

A catheter is a tube that drains urine from the bladder into a collection bag. The catheter gives the internal incision time to heal but meanwhile you may feel some discomfort. Urine may bypass (leak around) your catheter. If it leaks all the time or if there is no urine in the bag, let your nurse know. Before you leave the hospital, the nurse will show you how to care for your catheter.

Temperature Fluctuations

It may take a week for your body to regain its normal constant temperature. At times you may feel very cold and then very hot. It helps to lie on a towel to absorb perspiration when feeling hot.

Scrotal Swelling and Bruising

You will notice that your scrotal area is swollen and sweaty, with some bruising. The swelling will last for a couple of weeks. Sitting on a regular pillow can help alleviate discomfort. Showering frequently will help.

Mood Swings

Following surgery your emotions may be delicately balanced. As a result you may notice that you have rapid mood swings; tearful and sad one minute and then cheerful and relieved the next.

Tips to Help Avoid Problems After Surgery

Get Out of Bed

Usually, the day of surgery, a nurse will help you sit at the side of the bed. You may not feel very strong or steady at first, but you should progress to sitting in a chair later in the day.

To get out of bed, both in hospital and at home:

1. If the bed is electric, raise the head of the bed yourself or ask someone to do it for you.

2. Bend your knees and roll onto your side. This helps even with ordinary beds.

3. Swing your feet and legs over the edge of the bed. Bring your body to a sitting position.

4. Pause and take a few deep breaths before standing up.

5. While standing, pause again, breathe, then move to the chair.

Deep Breathing and Coughing

A physiotherapist or nurse will assist you with breathing exercises to help keep your lungs healthy. Deep breathing and coughing after surgery is very important, even if it causes you some discomfort keep your lungs healthy. Hold a pillow snugly over your incision when you cough and take deep breaths. You may be given a small device called an incentive spirometer to help you breathe deeply. The nurses will show you how to use it.

Pneumatic Stockings/Pressure Stockings

You may have special stockings on after surgery to improve circulation and help prevent blood clots while you are in bed. Pneumatic stockings are somewhat bulky "bubble pack" stockings attached to an air compressor. Pressure stockings are elastic stockings that look like heavy white nylons. These stockings are to be worn until you are walking several times a day.

Move Around In Bed

While you are in bed, be sure to change your position every 2 hours. Before moving, hold a small pillow over your incision(s). Bend your knees and roll from side to side. Bend and stretch your legs, feet, and toes every hour when you are awake. Exercising your legs and feet in bed helps your blood circulate.

Walk, Walk, Walk!

Once you can get up, you should begin to walk. Exercise helps circulation and healing and also relieves gas. You may need pain medication before you walk. Activity should be short and frequent, rather than over a long period of time. It is usual to need assistance to walk for the first time. Walk farther as you feel stronger and steadier on your feet.

Tips About Drinking Fluids and Eating

Surgery can upset your digestive system. Although you may feel thirsty, you must not eat or drink until your bowels are ready. Your urologist and nurses will ask you if you are "passing gas." This information lets them know whether your bowels are getting back to normal. As your bowels start working again, you will first be given small amounts of fluids, then a light diet, and finally regular food. Walking and fluids are very good for your digestive system.

Bowel Movements, Gas Pains, Constipation

It may take up to 5 days to have a bowel movement. To avoid gas pains and constipation, take small bites of food and chew well. Drink fluids once you can. Eat foods that you find easy to digest. And WALK!

Going Home

How Long Will I Be in Hospital?

Most men stay for 2 days. Some stay longer.

When Should I Start Planning for Discharge?

Ask questions about what to do after you are discharged right from the time of admission. Find out which matters you will see the urologist (your surgeon) about and when you can see your family physician. If you do not live in the city where you had your surgery, you will probably be in contact with your family physician more often, but will still need to follow up with your urologist at times.

Discuss the medication, care, and supplies you will need and who will help you. Some partners may be worried about providing care without help.

If you live alone, you may need visits from a home care nurse. She or he can be a resource if you have questions, especially about your catheter, incision, or pain control. Soon after surgery, discuss your concerns with your urologist and with the nurse who will help with discharge planning. Your local Prostate Cancer Support Group could be a source of information for you as well.

Any Tips for the Ride Home?

- Take your pain medication at least 30 minutes before leaving the hospital.

- You should not drive home.

- Wear a pair of pants that are loose around the waist and legs and that don't need a belt. This will help you feel more comfortable over your incision site(s). You may want to wear an incontinence pad, and put a waterproof protective pad on the seat of the car before you sit down.

- A pillow held over the abdomen may be helpful while riding in the car, as will adjusting the seat.

- You will still have a catheter, either attached to a small bag secured around your lower leg or to the larger drainage bag you used in the hospital. Be sure that whatever bag you are using is empty before leaving the hospital. If you have a large drainage bag, plan for a spot to hang it so that the top of the bag is not above the level of your penis. If you have a long drive home, have a container to empty urine from the small bag into, as well as a few extra incontinence pads.

You will probably feel tired and need to rest when you get home.

Discharge Checklist

Before you leave the hospital, you will be given a discharge checklist that your nurse will discuss with you. It will spell out information such as:

☐ activity restrictions (on work, lifting, driving)

_____

☐ medications

_____

☐ bladder control

_____

☐ nursing unit phone number

_____

☐ home care number

_____

☐ catheter care

_____

☐ date and time of catheter removal appointment

_____

☐ your next urologist appointment

_____

AFTER SURGERY, AT HOME

A radical prostatectomy is major surgery no matter which procedure has been performed. Give yourself time to recover. This can take a few months.

The following pages cover a wide range of topics to help you better understand what you can and cannot do, and when you need to contact your urologist or family physician. This information should help you manage your recovery at home.

Feeling Tired, Tired, Tired

"I feel like I've been hit by a truck." It is normal to feel very tired after surgery. Your energy will return, but it will take time. Most men feel better 4 to 6 weeks after surgery and return to work after 6 weeks. Let your body be your guide. Discuss any specific concerns with your urologist.

Feeling Emotional

Men have different feelings after surgery. You may have rapid mood swings. There may still be some fear or uncertainty about your recovery, and a feeling of lack of control. On the other hand there is relief that the cancer has been removed and that the surgery is over and you are now home. This emotional rollercoaster may continue for a while. Talk to people you are comfortable with and with your health professionals about how you are feeling. It is also important to share these feelings with your partner and other people close to you. Those men who met with a counsellor after surgery reported that they found it very helpful. Contact the Canadian Prostate Cancer Network for the most up-to-date information *http://www.cpcn.org*

Pain and Discomfort

Your family physician or urologist may suggest pain medication (analgesics) when you go home. Most men need analgesics for a about a week. Take analgesics 1/2 hour before activity and before going to bed. They usually take about 20 minutes to work. If your pain does not go away, call your family physician or urologist.

Physical Activity (first 6 weeks)

- No strenuous exercises
- No lifting more than 4 kg (10 lb)
- No snow shoveling, vacuuming, or pushing a lawn mower
- It is recommended that you do not drive while you have a catheter. After the catheter is removed, you can drive once you feel able.
- After the first week, you should become more active.
  - *Walking is excellent exercise. Start with short distances, increasing as you feel able.*
  - *Slowly start regular activities (housekeeping, other exercise) over 8 weeks. Do the activities that you enjoy the most, but be sure to take frequent rest periods.*

Care of Your Incision

You may go home from the hospital with a bandage or steri-strips over your incision(s). Keep your incision(s) clean and dry. A bandage is not needed if there is no drainage.

If you have a drain, a nurse will show you how to care for it before you go home.

If you go home with staples, a nurse or your family physician may remove them in about a week. After the staples are removed, steri-strips may be used on the incision. These will peel off.

It is common to be itchy around the incision(s). Try not to scratch. The incision area(s) may be sore. The discomfort will lessen with healing. You will see some swelling and/or bruising around the incision(s) that may last for weeks. In time, scar tissue will develop.

Notify your urologist if:

- you experience increased drainage or discharge from your incision area.
- the incision becomes red, puffy, or tender.
- the incision opens.

Bathing/Showering

You may take a shower whether you have steri-strips, staples, or a drain.

If you have a catheter, do not take a bath, only a shower.

Some men reported that frequent showering improved how they felt.

You can take a bath after the catheter, drain, and staples or steri-strips are removed.

After bathing or showering, carefully pat your incision dry with a clean towel.

Food and Fluids

Eat a well-balanced diet with fresh fruit, vegetables, protein, and dairy products.

Drink about 2 litres of fluid a day.

Avoiding caffeinated beverages may be helpful for your bladder.

Bowel Movements, Constipation

Your usual bowel movement schedule should resume within the first week. You may, however, become constipated. Constipation can result from either a low fluid intake, a diet low in fibre, pain medication, and inactivity, or a combination of these.

Do not strain to have a bowel movement as this causes pressure on your incision. You may need to take a stool softener to make bowel movements ("stools") easier to pass. It may also help to support your lower abdomen with your hands or a pillow while you are having a bowel movement.

The Catheter

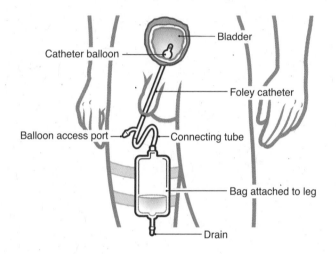

Bladder

Catheter balloon

Foley catheter

Balloon access port — Connecting tube

Bag attached to leg

Drain

You will have a catheter in place for 1 to 3 weeks, and maybe longer. The catheter will drain urine until your incision inside is healed. Your family physician or urologist will determine the best time to remove the catheter.

You will have two collection bags: a large one and a small one. The large bag hangs at the side of your bed or chair. To hang a bag, put a strong plastic clothes hanger under your mattress, then hang the bag on the hook. It is best to use the large bag at night. The small bag is used when you are walking. It is held to your leg with straps and fits under your clothing. If you find the leg straps uncomfortable, you can buy more comfortable cloth straps from a medical supplier.

What Can I Expect with the Catheter?

Here are the most common complaints men have about the catheter.

- Leakage of urine around the catheter is normal after surgery, caused by bladder spasms, kinked tubing, or constipation. Although inconvenient, leakage means that the incision inside (where the prostate was removed) is healing, and preventing any inside leakage of urine. An incontinence pad can protect your clothing. Protective pads can protect your furniture.

- Bladder spasms are uncomfortable contractions of the bladder muscle. The bladder may feel full and you may have a strong urge to urinate. If these spasms persist, contact your family physician or urologist, who may prescribe medication to help settle the bladder.

- Small numbers of blood clots in the tubing or bag are normal. Drink at least 1.5 litres of non-caffeinated, non-alcoholic liquid each day to help remove small clots.

- Small amounts of blood and mucous oozing around the catheter at the tip of the penis are normal. Keep the area clean. Close fitting underwear or an incontinence pad can help hold the catheter close to your body. This will stop the catheter from moving and making the penis sore. Put vaseline, Polysporin® or Neosporin® ointment (non-prescription) on the tip of the penis to help reduce irritation from the catheter tube.

- Bladder infections are uncommon.

Emptying the Drainage Bag

1. Empty your bag when it is half full, to avoid accidents!

2. Wash your hands.

3. To empty the drainage bag hold the bag over the toilet, loosen the clamp on the tubing at the bottom of the bag, and drain the urine into the toilet. You can also drain the urine into a container first (a large jar) and then empty the container into the toilet.

4. When you are finished, tighten the tubing.

5. Wipe the tip of the drainage tubing with an alcohol swab before putting it into "cap."

6. Wash your hands.

Cleaning the Drainage Bag and Tubing

The drainage bags must be cleaned to prevent odour.

1. Wash your hands.

2. Disconnect the catheter and attach it to an alternative bag.

3. Rinse the bag and tubing with cold water.

4. Fill the drainage bag with a solution of 2 parts vinegar to 3 parts water. (Some men find a turkey baster useful for putting this solution into the bag.)

5. Let the bag and solution sit for 30 minutes, then drain.

6. Rinse the bag with water and hang to dry.

7. Clean the cap and tubing with alcohol swabs.

8. Wash your hands.

Symptoms of a bladder infection:

Call your urologist or your family physician, or go to Emergency if you experience any of the following

- Chills & Fever (temperature greater than 38.5° C)
- An increase in mucous and/or sediment in the urine
- Dull pain over the kidney area
- No urine drainage from the catheter into the bag
- Increase in abdominal pain
- Blood clots or bright red urine
- Bladder spasms that do not go away.

Catheter Removal

Your family physician, nurse, or urologist will remove the catheter. Many men are fearful about this procedure but there should be minimal discomfort. The catheter slips out easily when the balloon that keeps the catheter in place is deflated (see page 40).

After the catheter is removed, you may have some urine leakage. Take an incontinence pad with you and use a protective pad on the car seat. Leakage or urinary incontinence (see page 45) can last from a few days to several months. Although the problem usually improves, it can be frustrating.

Some Urinary Symptoms after Catheter Removal

- No sensation of any urine in the bladder
- Frequency – the need to frequently go to the bathroom (more than 6 or 7 times in a 24-hour period)
- Nocturia – the need to go to the bathroom at night more than twice
- Urgency – the sudden need to urinate immediately
- Urge Incontinence – urine leakage when you feel a sudden need to urinate and can't make it to the bathroom on time
- Stress Incontinence – urine leakage when doing anything that causes pressure on the bladder. This includes coughing, sneezing, laughing, lifting, jogging, or passing gas.

Remember, these symptoms will improve with time and vary with each man.

On rare occasions, urine blockages (strictures) can occur. Call your urologist or family physician if:

- your urine stream gets weak
- you have to strain to start the stream
- your stream stops and starts
- you cannot pass your water at all.

Urinary Incontinence

Most men leak urine for a period of time following catheter removal, although the length of this time varies from person to person. Coping with incontinence is one of the concerns that men talk about after a radical prostatectomy. Knowing what to expect will help you cope with the inconvenience of leakage.

Initially, expect urinary incontinence for a few months. Most men regain bladder control by 3 to 6 months, though it may take longer for some.

Managing Leakage

- Be patient.
- Empty your bladder about every 2 to 4 hours.
- Do pelvic floor muscle exercises.
- Exercise regularly and maintain or reduce your weight. Being overweight can make stress incontinence worse.
- Drink plenty of fluids. Don't withhold fluids to prevent leakage because doing so may cause other problems that are more serious, such as infection or constipation.
- Keep bowels regular. Constipation may make incontinence worse.
- Learn to control the urge to empty your bladder (see page 47).
- Over time, you will gradually be able to increase the time between voiding.

Pelvic Floor Muscle Exercises

Pelvic floor muscle exercises may help to reduce urinary incontinence. Do NOT do the exercises if your catheter is still in place.

You may do the exercises sitting, standing, or lying down. Imagine you are trying to stop yourself from passing gas by squeezing the muscle around your anus. You should feel the anus muscle move while the buttocks, thighs, and stomach stay relaxed (without moving). If you are doing the exercise correctly, you should be able to feel, and if you look, to see, the base of your penis twitch, and contract inwards.

⇨ *SQUEEZE firmly for 5 to 10 seconds.*
⇨ *RELAX for 10 to 20 seconds.*
⇨ *REPEAT the contractions 12 to 20 times.*
⇨ *Do the exercises 3 times a day.*

The exercises are easy. If you find it difficult to isolate the right muscles, a physiotherapist or nurse who specializes in these exercises can explain how to do them correctly. Ask your health professional for information about who provides this service in your area. The nearest Prostate Cancer Support Group may have audiovisual materials in various formats to help you learn how to do these exercises.

When You Get the Urge to Urinate

- Stop what you are doing and stand still or sit down.
- Breathe slowly and relax.
- Concentrate on controlling the urge.
- Distraction may help. Count backward from 100.
- Do the pelvic floor muscle exercises 5 to 10 times.
- After the urge passes, try to delay voiding so that you are only emptying your bladder approximately every two hours.

A urology nurse, physiotherapist, or urologist can help you learn to control the urge to empty your bladder.

Incontinence Pads

There are a number of pads to choose from. Talk to a medical supplier or your home care nurse to discuss the best pad for you. Some of the different options made especially for men, are smallish pads called guards, larger disposable undergarments, or briefs in one-piece or two-piece systems. Protective pads for covering your bed and chair coverings are also available. You can buy these products in pharmacies or from medical suppliers. Some supplies may be available at large retail outlets. Discuss the options with your urology nurse.

Erectile Dysfunction (Problems Having Erections)

After a radical prostatectomy, many men are not able to have an erection. The nerves to the penis may be damaged or removed during surgery. For some men, erections will return, but they are different than before. The return of erections varies with age, health, and the specific surgery.

Removing the prostate, however, does not affect your hormone balance or sex drive. You may experience frustration if you have the desire to have sex but are unable to have an erection.

Manual or oral stimulation may produce a mild orgasm even in a flaccid penis, which can be encouraging in the early stages of recovery. This is referred to as a "dry" orgasm. There will be no release of semen with an orgasm because the prostate gland and seminal vesicles that produce semen have been removed. Such activity may also indicate beginning recovery of erectile function.

Erectile dysfunction can be difficult for men and their partners. Counselling can be helpful. Although many find this subject embarrassing, please discuss it with your urologist.

Penile Rehabilitation

If you experience erectile dysfunction, other resources may be helpful for you. These include different treatment options (pills, injections, vacuum devices, and penile implants) collectively referred to as penile rehabilitation. Treatments can start as soon as you and your partner are ready.

Follow-Up with Your Urologist

Report any problems mentioned in the information provided in this section. Keep a list of these concerns to discuss during your visit.

Even if you do not have any particular problems with your recovery, you will need to see your urologist on a regular basis. Regular PSA blood testing will be ordered. This testing will help to determine whether there is any further prostate cancer activity. If there is, additional treatment options will be discussed.

Back to Work

The usual time off work varies from person to person. Return only when YOU feel ready. Discuss this with your partner, urologist, or other health professional.

Your Partner/Family

The recovery time is stressful for those who care about you. Being non-communicative can lead to problems with your partner, who can be your best friend. Your recovery may be less stressful if you share what you are feeling. Finding opportunities for humour and laughter can help you both relieve stress for a period.

Partners and children may also feel the need for support and reassurance. Encourage them to talk to you, each other, and to a health professional. Psychologists and counselors are available at your local cancer facility. Attending Prostate Cancer Support Group meetings can be very helpful.

CLOSING WORDS

In this comprehensive guide we have included information that we hope will help you understand what to expect when undergoing a radical prostatectomy, as well as tips about managing BEFORE and AFTER your surgery. Your experience will not necessarily include all the events described.

   While a radical prostate surgery is a stressful experience, as is any surgery, the support of your loved ones and your health care team can assist you. Most men recover well and go on to experience a very good quality of life.

   Remember, become as informed as possible and be involved in discussions and plans regarding your care. Ask questions. Talk to your partner and family. Be prepared by getting fit and keeping a positive attitude!

RESOURCES

The men and their partners who met with us to share their experiences of radical prostatectomy stressed the importance of being well informed, but found that not all resources were reliable.

Because each person's experience is unique, a wide variety of resources are included in this guide. Those listed are recommended as reliable and useful sources of information based on both the input of participants as to what they found helpful, and on guidelines for reviewing websites. Discuss what you read with your health care professionals as well.

As the management of prostate cancer and prostate surgery will vary among physicians, urologists, hospitals, provinces, and countries, ask your urologist and other members of your health care team for specific resources they recommend.

Local Cancer Institute

The Cancer Institute that you attend for the diagnosis and management of your cancer should have a library with excellent information for your use.

Prostate Cancer Support Groups

Prostate Cancer Support Groups (PCSG) provide support and information to men and their partners. Those who have become involved with their local PCSG have reported that this experience was very helpful. Regularly scheduled meetings provide a forum for information exchange about prostate cancer and treatments, for facilitating contact with others who have had prostate cancer, as well as for opportunities for humour and friendship.

Ask your health care team for information about the your local PCSG near where you live. You can also contact the Canadian Cancer Society at *www.cancer.ca* to find the link to your local or provincial division to obtain contact information about your local PCSG. You can also call the Canadian Cancer Society at 1-888-939-3333.

Books

Goldenburg, S.L., & Thompson, I.M. (2001). *Intelligent patient guide to prostate cancer: All you need to know to take an active part in your treatment* (3rd Ed.) Vancouver, BC: Intelligent Patient Guides. ISBN 0-9696125-5-9.

A comprehensive, illustrated, self-help book for prostate cancer patients and their families. A clear step by step explanation of every aspect of prostate cancer gives patients the knowledge to take an active part in their treatment. Topics include: what prostate cancer is, reducing the risk of prostate cancer, detection, treatments, surgery, alternative therapies, and physical and psychological impact. The book also contains addresses and phone numbers of cancer treatment centres and support groups in Canada and the US.

McCormack, M., & Saad, F. (2004). *Understanding prostate cancer.* Montreal, QC: Rogers Media.

Written by two reputable Canadian urologists, this guide provides a simple, practical and yet complete overview of prostate cancer for men and their families and presents strategies for managing prostate cancer. Available free in French and English from ProCure Alliance - *http://www.procure.ca.*

Strum, B., & Pogliano, D. (2002). *A primer on prostate cancer: The empowered patient's guide.* (2nd Ed.) Florida: The Life Extension Foundation. ISBN 0-9658777-6-0

Written for men who have been diagnosed with prostate cancer. This resource outlines a strategy of disease management designed to help patients, their loved ones, and their doctors to optimize outcomes. A current, comprehensive and unbiased resource for prostate cancer patients, caregivers, partners, and physicians.

Other Material

Our Voice – a quarterly Canadian publication for men who have been diagnosed with prostate cancer. For a free subscription, go online to
http://www.ourvoiceinprostatecancer.com
or send your name and address to:
400 McGill St., 3rd Floor, Montreal QC H2Y 2G1,
Tel.: (514) 397-8833.

The Source: Your guide to better bladder control.
Available at www.canadiancontinence.ca/pdf/The-Source.pdf

Video

Prostate cancer: Conquering the fear. Newmarket Prostate Cancer Support Group (2002). Newmarket, ON: Newmarket Prostate Cancer Support Group, Rogers Television and AstraZeneca (includes graphic images of the actual surgery).

Reliable Websites

Canadian Cancer Society
http://www.cancer.ca

Canadian Continence Foundation
http://www.canadiancontinence.ca

The Canadian Health Network
http://www.canadian-health-network.ca

Canadian Prostate Cancer Network
http://www.cpcn.org

The Canadian Prostate Health Council
http://canadian-prostate.com

The Canadian Urological Association
http://www.cua.org

The Canadian Urological Oncology Group
http://www.cuog.org

Health Canada:
http://www.hc-sc.gc.ca/

ProCure Alliance:
http://www.procure.ca

Prostate Cancer Information (Health Canada and the Department of Urology, Dalhousie University)
http://www.caprostate.com

Prostate Cancer Research Foundation of Canada
http://www.prostatecancer.ca

The "New" Prostate Cancer Infolink
http://www.prostatecancerinfolink.net/

The Prostate Centre Clinic Toronto
http://www.prostatecentre.ca/resources_clinic.html

Prostate Info
http://www.prostateinfo.com

Public Health Agency of Canada, Centre for Chronic Disease Prevention and Control
http://www.phac-aspc.gc.ca/

Rapid Access Clinic, Prostate Cancer Institute
http://www.prostatecalgary.com/

Safeway Father's Day Walk/Run for Prostate Cancer
http//www.fathersdayrun.ca/home/

Urology Nurses of Canada
http://www.unc.org

You are not alone!
http://www.yananow.net/

YOUR NOTES

IMPORTANT
TELEPHONE
NUMBERS

Cancer Treatment Centre: _____

Home Care: _____

Home Care Nurse: _____

Hospital: _____

  Pre Admission Clinic (PAC): _____

  Urology Unit at the Hospital: _____

Medical Care Supplier: _____

Pharmacy: _____

Physiotherapist: _____

Physician (Family): _____

Prostate Cancer Support Group: _____

Urologist: _____

Urology Nurse: _____

Other: _____